INTRODUCTION:

The Importance of Nutrition in the NICU Knowing the NICU A specialized medical facility called the Neonatal Intensive Care Unit (NICU) is meant to treat premature and seriously ill neonates. Specialized care and support are necessary for infants admitted to the NICU because they frequently confront unique problems. These difficulties could consist of Premature Birth: Babies born before 37 weeks of pregnancy may have organs and systems that are not fully developed, which puts them at risk for issues. Low Birth Weight: Many newborns in the intensive care unit have low birth weights, affecting how well they can grow, fight infections, and control their body temperature. Medical Conditions: Serious medical intervention and surveillance are necessary for infections, congenital anomalies, and respiratory distress syndrome. A multidisciplinary team of medical specialists, including neonatologists, nurses, respiratory therapists, and dietitians, staffs the state-of-the-art NICU. They offer complete care to promote these vulnerable newborns' development and well-being. Summary of the Function of Nutrition in Development Nutrition is the foundation of newborn care in the NICU. It is critical for their overall health, development, and growth. Meeting the dietary demands of NICU infants can substantially impact their short- and long-term results, as their needs differ greatly from those of full-term, healthy newborns. Vital Functions of Diet in the Development of NICUs: Encouraging Growth: Sufficient nourishment ensures that neonates receive the right amount of weight and develop at the right pace. This is critical for their overall growth and ensuring they are ready to leave the hospital. Supporting Organ Development: The development of key organs, such as the brain, lungs, and digestive system, is aided by essential nutrients. Improving

Immune Function: Eating a healthy diet strengthens the immune system, which helps shield NICU babies from diseases and infections. Enhancing Neurodevelopmental Outcomes: Research has shown a connection between improved neurological and cognitive development and improved neurodevelopment, which can have long-term impacts on behavior and learning.

Encouraging Healing and Recuperation: Adequate nourishment promotes tissue healing and healing in infants recuperating from operations or medical procedures. The goal of the book "Healthy Eating for Kids: A Complete Guide to NICU Nutrition for Babies" is to serve as an all-

HEALTHY EATING FOR KIDS

A Complete Guide to NICU Nutrition for Babies

TABLE OF CONTENTS

encompassing reference for medical professionals, parents, and other caregivers involved in NICU baby care. The book seeks to: Educate and give comprehensive information regarding the special dietary requirements of neonates in intensive care units (NICUs) and the range of feeding techniques that are employed to address these requirements. Support: Provide helpful advice on feeding methods, growth tracking, and typical nutrition-related issues in NICUs. Inspire: To provide hope and encouragement to families facing the NICU journey, as well as to share real stories and experiences from parents and healthcare professionals. Advocate: Stress the importance of a multidisciplinary approach to NICU care, as well as the need for families and medical professionals to work together. Through this book, we want to equip parents and other caregivers with the knowledge and resources necessary to make wise choices regarding their child's diet. We can guarantee that newborns in the intensive care unit (NICU) have the finest start in life possible by emphasizing optimum nutrition, which will establish the groundwork for their healthy growth and development.

CHAPTER 1: THE BASICS OF NICU NUTRITION

Crucial nutritional requirements for sick and premature infants Compared to healthy, full-term neonates, premature and critically ill infants have different and more intense dietary requirements. These needs must be met for their long-term development, growth, and survival. Important nutritional elements: Calories: To maintain their quick growth and development, premature newborns need more calories per kilogram of body weight than full-term infants. Depending on the infant's age, weight, health, and rate of growth, different calorie requirements may apply. Proteins are essential for muscle and organ development, tissue healing, and growth. Premature babies require more protein to maintain their faster growth and make up for any protein deficiencies brought on by disease or preterm birth. Glucose: For babies in the NICU, carbohydrates are the main source of energy. Sufficient consumption of carbohydrates is necessary to meet the body's high energy needs and keep the body from converting proteins into energy. Lipids: The development of the brain depends on fats, particularly long-chain polyunsaturated fatty acids (LCPUFAs) like DHA and ARA, which offer concentrated energy. vital for the neurological system's growth as well as the absorption of fat-soluble vitamins (A, D, E, and K). Minerals and Vitamins: Phosphorus and calcium are essential for bone growth and mineralization. Iron is required for hemoglobin synthesis and anemia prevention. The immune system and bone health are supported by vitamin D. Additional micronutrients: These include magnesium, copper, and zinc, all of which are essential for different metabolic processes. Fluids: Because of their immature kidneys and increased body surface area compared to weight, preterm newborns are more susceptible to fluid imbalances, so it's important to maintain appropriate hydration. Variations Nutrition: A Comparison of Full-Term and Preterm Because of their earlier developmental stage and the difficulties they encounter, premature babies have different dietary needs than full-term babies. Important variations include the following: Rate of Growth: During the early postnatal period, preterm newborns grow faster than full-term infants, and they need more calories and nutrients to maintain this accelerated growth. The gastrointestinal tract's function Preterm babies' less developed digestive systems make it more difficult for them to properly digest and absorb nutrients. Common problems include delayed stomach emptying, immature enzyme synthesis, and abnormal motility of the gut. Stores of nutrients: Because they spend less time in utero, preterm babies have smaller reserves of important nutrients, including iron, calcium, and fat-soluble vitamins. To meet their needs, they rely increasingly on postnatal nourishment. Preterm babies have higher metabolic needs because they must grow, recover, and maintain body temperature. This means that their dietary needs are higher. Immune System: Because of their immature immune systems, preterm babies are more susceptible to infections and require nutrients to boost immunity. Typical nutritional obstacles in the NICU There are various obstacles to meeting the dietary requirements of newborns in NICUs: Intolerance to Food: Feeding intolerance may be indicated by symptoms like diarrhea, vomiting, and distension in the abdomen. Management techniques for feeding intolerance include using medication, modifying formulations, and tweaking feeding quantities and rates are among the management techniques for feeding intolerance. Enterocolitis that necrotizes (NEC) is a dangerous intestinal illness that primarily affects premature infants. It can complicate nutritional treatment and be fatal. The use of human milk and the cautious progression of enteral feeding are examples of preventive strategies. Sepsis and Infections: Nutritional management can be made more difficult by infections, which can change nutrient use and raise metabolic needs. Reflux of the stomach (GER): Preterm babies frequently get GER, which can lead to pain and feeding issues. Medication, feed thickeners, and placement techniques are all part of management. Parenteral Nutrition (PN) Hazards: Long-term PN usage is associated with infection, liver damage, and metabolic abnormalities. It's critical to monitor closely and switch to enteral feedings as soon as feasible. Monitoring and adjusting for growth: To guarantee optimal growth, measurements of weight, length, head circumference, and nutritional intake must be made regularly. The infant's progress and tolerance require regular adjustments to the nutritional recommendations.

CHAPTER 2: BREAST MILK: THE GOLD STANDARD

Breast milk's advantages for NICU babies Breast milk is widely regarded as the optimal form of nutrition for infants, with its advantages being particularly noticeable for neonates receiving care in the Neonatal Intensive Care Unit (NICU). Breast milk offers several benefits to newborns in the intensive care unit, especially those delivered prematurely: Optimal Nutrition: Specifically formulated to meet the needs of infants, breast milk offers the ideal proportion of proteins, lipids, carbs, vitamins, and minerals. Immune Support: Breast milk, which is high in antibodies, white blood cells, and other immune-stimulating substances, aids in defending NICU babies against infections and diseases. Digestive Health: Breast milk helps an infant's digestive tract mature and encourages the growth of beneficial gut flora. Benefits for Neurodevelopment: Elements such as long-chain polyunsaturated fatty acids (LCPUFAs) found in breast milk are essential for cognitive development and brain growth. Bonding: A baby's emotional growth depends on the mother and child's emotional relationship being strengthened through breastfeeding or the provision of breast milk. How to Pump and Store Breast Milk Direct breastfeeding may not be possible for NICU mothers at first. Breastfeeding and conserving breast milk have become necessary routines. Pumping: To develop and sustain a milk supply, mothers should try to pump every two to three hours. Method: Increasing efficiency can be achieved by using a high-quality electric breast pump. To avoid infection, pumping equipment must be sterilized, and hands must be cleaned properly. Keeping: Containers: Use milk storage bags or clean, BPA-free containers. Labeling: Make sure the date and time of expression are written on each container. Freezing and Refrigeration: You can keep freshly expressed breast milk in the freezer for up to six months or in the refrigerator for up to four days. To maintain the quality of milk, defrost and warm according to the directions. Enhancing Breast Milk with Extra Nutrients Even though breast milk has a lot of nutrients, preterm babies frequently require extra help to support their quick development and growth. This is the role of fortification. Why Fortify? Compared to what breast milk alone can offer, premature babies have greater needs for calories, protein, calcium, phosphorus, and other nutrients. How to strengthen: To increase the nutritional value of expressed breast milk, human milk fortifiers (HMF) are added. Before feeding, these fortifiers—which come in liquid or powder form—are combined with the milk. Observation and Modification: Healthcare professionals keep a careful eye on the baby's development and biochemical markers to modify the fortification as necessary to guarantee the child gets enough nourishment without experiencing any imbalances. Parents and other caregivers can optimize the advantages of breast milk and offer NICU infants the greatest start in life by being aware of and putting these strategies into practice.

CHAPTER 3: FORMULA FEEDING IN THE NICU

Formula Types for Sick and Preterm Infants Although formula feeding becomes necessary in certain instances, breast milk is often the preferred source of nutrition for babies in the intensive care unit. Formulas used in the NICU are specifically created to cater to the peculiar dietary requirements of ill and premature infants. Infant Formulas for Preterm: High-Calorie Formulas: Compared to regular infant formulas, these formulas offer more calories per ounce, which helps premature newborns grow at the proper rates. Enhanced Nutrient Formulas: These are designed to provide more protein, vitamins, and minerals—like calcium and phosphorus—that are essential for the development of strong bones. Formulas for Hydrolyzed Proteins: Partially or extensively hydrolyzed: The proteins in these formulas are reduced in size to smaller peptides or amino acids, which facilitates simpler absorption and digestion for babies with developing digestive systems. Compound Formulas: Amino Acid-Based: These formulas, which contain amino acids—the most basic form of protein—are used for children with severe allergies or intolerances to lower the likelihood of allergic reactions. Particular Mixtures: Disease-specific formulas are created for certain medical diseases, such as severe gastrointestinal problems or metabolic disorders. Use of Formula Indications In the NICU, formula feeding may be recommended in the following situations: Insufficient Breast Milk Supply: When a baby's nutritional needs are not met by the mother's milk supply, Maternal health concerns: Disorders that make breastfeeding inappropriate, such as infections, drug use, or other medical conditions, Infant medical illnesses: Certain infants require specific formula feeding due to illnesses such as galactosemia or certain metabolic problems. Feeding Intolerance: Specialized formulas may be necessary for infants who are unable to tolerate breast milk, even when it is fortified. Nutritional supplementation: when a person requires more calories or a certain nutrient than what breast milk or donor milk can offer. Safe Formula Administration and Preparation For NICU newborns' health and well-being, formula preparation and administration must be done safely. Sanitization and personal care: Equipment: To avoid contamination, all bottles, nipples, and feeding apparatus should be completely disinfected before use. Hand Hygiene: Before handling formula and feeding supplies, caregivers must properly wash their hands. Creating and Blending the Formula Follow the directions: To guarantee the right concentration and nutrient content, always follow the manufacturer's instructions while producing and mixing the formula. Water Quality: When mixing the solution, use sterile or suitably treated water, especially in areas where the water quality is dubious. Keeping and Managing: Refrigeration: If the prepared formula is not used right away, it should be refrigerated and thrown out after 24 hours. Warming: The formula can be made more comfortable by submerging the bottle in a warm water container. Microwaves should not be used since they can produce hot spots that could burn an infant's mouth. Feeding Procedures: Feeding Cues: Pay attention to your baby's cues about when to eat and when they're satisfied. Paced feeding can help avoid overfeeding and lower the risk of aspiration by letting the baby eat at their speed. Observation: Keep a close eye on the baby's tolerance to the formula and note any indications of discomfort, allergic reactions, or digestive problems. Caregivers can ensure that newborns in the NICU receive the nourishment they need safely and efficiently by being aware of the many types of formulas, their indications, and the best procedures for preparation and administration. This all-encompassing strategy supports these infants' sensitive growth, development, and general health.

CHAPTER 4: PARENTERAL NUTRITION

Parenteral nutrition: what is it? Parenteral nutrition, or PN, is the intravenous delivery of nutrients without any interaction with the gastrointestinal (GI) system. It delivers vital nutrients, including amino acids, carbohydrates, lipids, vitamins, and minerals, straight into the bloodstream. When a baby's digestive system is too immature or undeveloped to support enteral (oral or tube) feeding, PN is employed. Administration and Indications When a baby in the NICU is unable to get enough nutrition through their mouth because of GI abnormalities, severe prematurity, or recuperation from surgery, PN is recommended. PN is painstakingly made and customized to fit the unique requirements of every baby. Parts: Amino acids provide the necessary protein for tissue repair and growth. Dextrose: Provides energy-giving carbs. Lipids are fatty acids that are necessary for energy and brain development. Vitamins, trace elements, and electrolytes support a variety of metabolic processes as well as general health. Management: For safe and efficient nutrient delivery, PN is usually given via a central venous catheter. To avoid difficulties, it is imperative to continuously monitor blood glucose levels, electrolyte balances, and fluid balance. Making the Switch from Parenteral to Enteral Nutrition A crucial stage in NICU care is the switch from parenteral nutrition to enteral feeding, which denotes increased GI function and preparedness for more naturally occurring nutrition. Gradual Introduction: To gauge tolerance, enteral feeds are gradually added, commencing at modest quantities. Monitoring: Careful observation is kept of the baby's development, feces habits, and feeding tolerance. Weaning PN: To promote normal GI development and lower the risk of PN-associated problems, PN is gradually lowered as enteral feeding rises until the newborn can get full nourishment enterally. The infant's growth is supported during this gradual transition, which also gets them ready for long-term health and ultimate discharge.

CHAPTER 5: ENTERAL FEEDING METHODS

Orogastric, Gastrostomy, and Nasogastric Tubes Enteral feeding is the process of giving food directly to the stomach or intestines through feeding tubes. Nasogastric tubes (NGs) are often used for short-term feeding in neonatal intensive care units (NICUs). NG tubes are inserted through the nose and into the stomach. Orogastric (OG) tubes are an alternative to NG tubes in cases where nasal access is not practical. OG tubes are similar to NG tubes but are put through the mouth. Gastrostomy tubes, often known as G-tubes, are surgically inserted through the abdominal wall into the stomach to provide long-term nutrition. Starting and

Progressing with Enteral Feeds Starting the Feeds: Enteral feedings are started gradually, frequently with small amounts of specialty formula or breast milk. Usually, a pump is used to continually provide the first feeds to reduce the possibility of feeding intolerance. Advancing Feeds: The volume and concentration of feeds are gradually increased as tolerance is established. To replicate typical eating patterns and encourage digestive development, switching to intermittent bolus feeds may also take place. Handling Intolerance to Food Changes in stool patterns, vomiting, or distension in the abdomen can all be signs of feeding intolerance. Among the methods for handling feeding intolerance are:

Slow Advancement: To give the baby's digestive system time to adjust, meals should be introduced gradually and carefully. Changing the type or concentration of the formula or fortifier used is known as "adjusting feed composition." Positioning: To minimize reflux and enhance gastric emptying, keep the baby upright both during and after feedings. Monitoring and Interventions: Keeping an eye out for indicators of intolerance regularly and acting quickly to make any necessary modifications to the feeding schedule or seek out extra medical care. Healthcare professionals can support the growth and nutritional requirements of NICU infants by carefully controlling enteral feeding techniques, which will facilitate a more seamless transition to full enteral nutrition.

CHAPTER 6: KEY NUTRIENTS FOR NICU BABIES

Carbohydrates, Fats, and Proteins Proteins: As the building blocks of tissues, organs, and muscles, proteins are essential for the growth and development of neonates in intensive care units. A higher protein intake is necessary for preterm babies' quick growth and healing. To satisfy their demands, high-quality, quickly digestible protein sources are crucial. For newborns in the intensive care unit, carbohydrates are their main energy source. The most basic type of carbohydrate, glucose, is essential for both general energy production and brain function. Giving the body enough carbs guarantees that it will use the proteins for development instead of energy. Fats: Fats are essential for brain development and provide a concentrated source of energy. Neural development and general growth require essential fatty acids, especially long-chain polyunsaturated fatty acids (LCPUFAs) like DHA and ARA. Additionally, fats help the fat-soluble vitamins (A, D, E, and K) absorb better. Minerals and vitamins Minerals and vitamins are essential for many metabolic reactions as well as general health. Calcium and phosphorus are essential for bone mineralization and development. Preterm children, who are deprived of the latter stages of in-utero bone building, are especially in need of these minerals. Iron: Iron is essential for the blood's ability to carry oxygen and is needed for the synthesis of hemoglobin and the prevention of anemia. The immune system and bone health are supported by vitamin D. To promote general growth and avoid rickets, adequate amounts are required. Additional Micronutrients: Immune system performance, enzymatic processes, and general growth and development depend on zinc, copper, magnesium, and other trace elements. Balance of electrolytes and hydration. It's crucial to keep NICU babies' electrolyte balance and fluid levels stable. They are more vulnerable to fluid imbalances because of their underdeveloped kidneys and higher body surface area in comparison to their weight. Hydration: Maintaining a healthy fluid intake helps with general metabolic processes and guards against dehydration. Electrolytes: Nerve function, muscle activity, and the preservation of acid-base balance all depend on sodium, potassium, chloride, and bicarbonate. Preventing imbalances and maintaining ideal levels need periodic monitoring and changes. Healthcare professionals may support NICU infants' growth, development, and general health while also providing them with the best start in life by carefully controlling these essential nutrients.

Monitoring growth parameters It's critical to track NICU infants' growth to evaluate their general health and development. Important growth metrics consist of the following: Weight: Regular weighing helps monitor an infant's developmental rate and nutritional status. Gaining weight steadily is a sign that you are eating well. Length: Measuring a baby's length may reveal information about their general development and linear growth. Head circumference: This measurement provides information about general health and nutritional status, as well as brain growth and neurological development. Analyzing Laboratory Data Lab tests are essential for tracking the health and nutritional status of newborns in the intensive care unit. Notable laboratory findings consist of the following: Blood glucose levels: Keeping an eye on blood sugar levels will help control energy balance and identify high or low blood sugar. Electrolytes: To maintain fluid and electrolyte balance, regular measurements of sodium, potassium, chloride, and bicarbonate are necessary. Complete Blood Count (CBC): This examination aids in the diagnosis of infections, anemia, and general health. Nutrient Levels: Ensuring that infants obtain enough nourishment is done by measuring the levels of vital nutrients such as calcium, phosphorus, iron, and vitamins. Adapting Diet Plans in Light of Development Dietary programs need to be flexible, adjusting to the NICU babies' evolving needs and stages of growth. Important things to think about are: Examining Growth Trends: Nutritional intake modifications are guided by a routine evaluation of test results and growth parameters. Caloric Requirements: As babies develop, their calorie requirements rise, requiring changes to nutritional concentrations and feeding amounts. Resolving shortages: Ensuring optimum growth and development requires identifying and resolving nutrient shortages through diet or supplementation. By regularly monitoring and evaluating growth, healthcare professionals can adjust nutrition strategies to provide the best outcomes for NICU infants.

CHAPTER 8: ADDRESSING COMMON FEEDING CHALLENGES

Intolerance to Certain Foods and Acid Reflux

In the NICU, feeding intolerance is a frequent problem that frequently presents as vomiting, diarrhea, or distension of the abdomen. Handling lactose intolerance entails:

Slow Advancement: Increasing feed amounts gradually will help the baby's digestive system adjust.

Feeding Methods: To reduce pain and reflux, use timed feeding and keep the baby upright both during and after feedings.

Another common problem is gastroesophageal reflux disease (GER), which causes the stomach's contents to reflux back into the esophagus. GER management entails:

Thickened Feeds: You can lessen reflux episodes by thickening your food with rice cereal or commercial thickeners.

Medication: Proton pump inhibitors and H2 blockers are examples of drugs that may be prescribed in severe situations.

Enterocolitis that necrotizes (NEC)

The severe and sometimes fatal illness known as necrotizing enterocolitis (NEC) is characterized by intestinal inflammation and infection. Among the management and preventative techniques are:

Breast Milk: Using donor or breast milk, which has protective qualities and is easier to digest.

Probiotics: Giving probiotics to support a balanced population of gut flora.

Cautious Feeding: Start feeding gradually and keep an eye out for any indications of NEC to act quickly.

Sensitivities and Allergies

NICU babies can be allergic to or sensitive to specific proteins or ingredients in their meals. To deal with these, one must:

Hypoallergenic Formulas: For infants with protein allergies, use hydrolyzed or amino acid-based formulas.

Elimination diets: To determine if symptoms improve for breastfeeding infants, mothers may need to cut common allergens like dairy and soy from their diet.

Healthcare professionals can enhance the nutritional outcomes and general health of neonatal intensive care unit (NICU) newborns by proactively addressing these common feeding problems.

CHAPTER 9: THE ROLE OF PARENTS IN NICU NUTRITION

NICU Support for Breastfeeding Mothers, in particular, is very important when it comes to NICU feeding. To support nursing in the NICU, access to lactation consultants, who can assist moms in creating and sustaining a milk supply by direct breastfeeding when it is feasible, is known as lactation support. Touch of Skin to Skin: promoting "kangaroo care," which involves holding the baby close to the mother to increase milk production and fortify the mother-child attachment. Including Parents in Decisions About Feeding Parental involvement in feeding decisions gives them authority and guarantees that their preferences and worries are taken into account. Education: teaching new parents the advantages of breastfeeding, the nutritional requirements of their infant, and the rationale behind particular feeding techniques. Collaboration: Promoting a collaborative relationship between healthcare practitioners and families by encouraging parents to participate in daily care routines and decision-making processes. Family support on an emotional level For parents, being in the NICU can be extremely taxing. Supporting someone emotionally is essential. Therapy Services: Providing parents with access to support groups and therapy to assist them in dealing with stress, worry, and a sense of powerlessness. Communication: keeping lines of communication open, sincere, and caring to inform and include parents in their child's care. Staff members in the NICU can assist parents in playing a crucial role in their child's nutrition and general well-being by aggressively encouraging breastfeeding, including parents in feeding decisions, and offering emotional support. In addition to improving the child's health, this involvement strengthens the link between parents and child and gives families confidence during difficult times.

CHAPTER 10: MULTIDISCIPLINARY APPROACH TO NICU NUTRITION

Functions of the Medical Group Comprehensive care for preterm and ill infants is ensured by a multidisciplinary approach to NICU nutrition. Important roles consist of: Neonatologists manage medical care and make important decisions about dietary planning and treatments. Dietitians: Focus on creating and modifying dietary regimens to suit each baby's unique requirements. Nurses: Give feedings, keep an eye on a baby's reactions, and give parents practical care and education. Lactation consultants encourage breastfeeding and assist mothers in expressing and storing their milk. Pharmacists: handle parenteral nutrition solutions, prepare them, and keep an eye out for drug interactions. Working together and communicating An effective multidisciplinary approach requires effective collaboration and communication. Regular Meetings: Hold daily or weekly multidisciplinary team meetings to discuss each baby's development, dietary requirements, and any changes to their care plans.

Common Documentation: utilizing shared electronic health records to ensure that everyone on the team participates in the treatment plan and has access to the most recent facts. Case Studies and Triumphant Narratives Presenting case studies and achievements might draw attention to the following advantages of a multidisciplinary approach: Personalized Care: Case studies can show how cooperatively created customized nutrition plans have significantly improved the health and growth of newborns. Testimonials from parents: Parent success stories highlight the benefits of all-encompassing, team-based care for both their child's growth and their own NICU stay. Better results for newborns and their families can be achieved by the healthcare team by using a multidisciplinary approach to provide holistic, well-coordinated care that covers all NICU nutrition-related issues.

CHAPTER 11: LONG-TERM OUTCOMES AND FOLLOW-UP

Early Nutrition's Effect on Long-Term Health For preterm and ill infants, early feeding in the NICU has a significant influence on long-term health outcomes. Sufficient nutrition during infancy promotes healthy growth, cognitive development, and immune system performance. Infants who receive enough nutrition are more likely to grow up with better general health, fewer developmental delays, and improved cognitive outcomes.

Making sure babies have the proper nutrition balance throughout their formative months can lower their lifetime risk of developing chronic illnesses, including obesity, diabetes, and cardiovascular disease. Making the transition to oral feeding For infants in the NICU, switching from tube feeding to oral feeding is a big milestone. This procedure includes: The evaluation of the infant's coordination in sucking, swallowing, and breathing—essential skills for safe oral feeding—is known as the readiness assessment. Slow Introductory: To guarantee sufficient nutrition, start with modest oral feeds while maintaining tube feedings. Parental Involvement: providing parents with information and opportunities to learn about feeding their infant to foster a sense of confidence in their abilities to do so. After-discharge Nutritional support and follow-up care Follow-up treatment is necessary after discharge to guarantee continued development and growth. This comprises Frequent check-ups: tracking development milestones, growth parameters, and general health. Nutritional guidance includes introducing solid foods to parents, as well as continuing to support and educate them about healthy nutrition. Referrals to specialists: If necessary, refer patients with feeding or developmental issues to specialists such as pediatric nutritionists, occupational therapists, or speech therapists. Healthcare professionals can contribute to NICU graduates' well-being and potential achievement by emphasizing long-term outcomes and providing comprehensive follow-up care.

CHAPTER 12: INNOVATIONS IN NICU NUTRITION

Developments in Food Technologies The administration and supply of nutrients to premature and unwell infants have been improved through recent advancements in feeding technologies, which have completely changed NICU nutrition. Human Milk Fortification Systems: Precise and constant supplementation, according to the individual requirements of each baby, is ensured by automated systems that fortify breast milk with vital nutrients, including protein, minerals, and vitamins. Enteral feeding devices: State-of-the-art feeding tubes and pumps minimize the risk of feeding intolerance and maximize nutritional absorption by enabling precise control over feeding amounts and rates. Parenteral Nutrition Formulations: Enhanced parenteral nutrition solutions offer well-rounded nutrition while lowering the risk of side effects such as infections and liver damage. Investigations into Nutritional Interventions Novel nutritional strategies that enhance outcomes for NICU newborns are still being investigated by ongoing research. Studies on the gut microbiome: looking into how the gut microbiota affects immunity, digestion, and general health, with possible applications to the creation of probiotic treatments. Studying the ideal dietary ratios and compositions to promote long-term health outcomes, neurodevelopment, and growth. Nutritional Supplements: Investigating whether specific nutrients or supplements can improve neurodevelopmental outcomes or lessen problems like necrotizing enterocolitis (NEC). Prospects for NICU Nutrition in the Future The future directions for NICU nutrition aim to further individualize care and improve results. Customizing diet regimens to meet each person's unique genetic, metabolic, and nutritional requirements is known as precision nutrition. Early Intervention Programs: To reduce long-term health risks and support ideal growth and development, early dietary interventions are put into place. Technology Integration: By predicting nutritional requirements based on real-time data and optimizing feeding regimens, artificial intelligence and data analytics are used. Healthcare professionals may continue to improve NICU nutrition and, ultimately, the health and quality of life for infants born prematurely or with complicated medical conditions.

CHAPTER 13: PERSONAL STORIES AND EXPERIENCES

Parent Testimonials Parents of newborns in the NICU frequently talk about their emotional journeys, emphasizing the difficulties and successes they encounter. These testimonies offer a very intimate perspective on the vital role that diet plays in their infant's healing and development. Parents describe the anguish of witnessing their small children struggle, as well as the comfort and hope they experienced when their children grew stronger due to a healthy diet. They also stress how the NICU staff's important instruction and assistance enabled parents to take an active role in their baby's care. Medical professionals' experiences The NICU's medical staff observes the revolutionary effects of feeding on newborn health. Their experiences demonstrate the commitment, knowledge, and empathy needed to handle the difficulties of NICU care. Providers discuss their experiences creating individualized diet programs, resolving feeding issues, and commemorating family anniversaries. These stories emphasize the cooperation between the parents and the medical staff and show how crucial a multidisciplinary approach is to providing the best care possible for NICU babies. Narratives of NICU Alums Resilience and the long-term advantages of early dietary interventions are demonstrated through the experiences of NICU graduates. These narratives frequently feature important developmental turning points, including first words, steps, and academic success, showing the benefits of careful nutritional management.

NICU alumni and their families frequently go on to become leaders in the field of neonatal health, sharing their personal stories to encourage and uplift others going through similar difficulties. In summary, nourishing optimism for the future Summary of Important Points: The essential elements of NICU nutrition have been covered in this book, including the role of parents and medical teams, the significance of breast milk and formula feeding, and how to manage feeding difficulties.

Motivation for Families and Those Who Care: Recall that you are not traveling this path alone, but with families and caregivers. NICU babies are incredibly resilient and strong, and they may grow and develop to amazing heights if given the correct care and nourishment. Additional support resources: Families are advised to get in touch with pediatric nutritionists, lactation consultants, and NICU support groups for continuing assistance. Resources that offer more community and direction include instructional websites, internet forums, and local support groups. This chapter aims to provide hope, inspiration, and useful guidance to families traveling the difficult but rewarding journey of NICU nutrition by sharing these personal stories and experiences.

CONCLUSION

The book "Healthy Eating for Kids: A Complete Guide to NICU Nutrition for Babies" ends with a contemplation on how important nutrition is to NICU babies' journeys. We have examined the challenges of giving unwell and premature babies the best nutrition throughout this book, highlighting the significant influence on their long-term health, development, and growth. Every chapter has emphasized the value of a multidisciplinary approach, from comprehending the particular dietary requirements of NICU babies to managing feeding difficulties, including intolerance and reflux. We have honored the accomplishments and fortitude of NICU graduates and their families, being moved by their tales of triumphing over hardship with the help of committed medical staff. Future developments in feeding technology, studies on nutritional therapies, and the incorporation of individualized care strategies will all contribute to the ongoing evolution of the field of NICU nutrition. It is evidence of the commitment of medical professionals, the resilience of families, and the potential for ongoing advancement in neonatal care. This book should help parents, caregivers, and medical professionals feel more informed, wise, and hopeful. I believe it will be a useful tool and a source of inspiration for families navigating the difficult but rewarding path of NICU nutrition, helping to maintain the health and well-being of our tiniest and most tenacious patients in the process.